Stress Explained

Stress Overview, Causes, Types, Management, Prevention, Common Stressors, History, Effects, Dealing with Stress – Related Problems and Much More!

By Frederick Earlstein

Copyrights and Trademarks

Disclaimer and Legal Notice

Foreword

There is no way we can have full control of everything that happens to us during our lifetime but we do have the ability to regulate the way we think and feel about the situations and event we face. None of us are born with manuals to tell us how to lead our lives, we go by intuition, tradition and common sense, but we definitely are twinned with stress the minute we are greeted by the world. It is as if stress was just standing on the sidelines waiting for our emergence and once we pop out of the confines of our serenely, tranquil world, we are handed the invisible energy of stress.

Stress it is everyone's inferno. It bedevils our minds. It disrupts and ignites our nights, as it upends our equilibrium and modifies our chemistry. It was once meant to save us from living in the wilderness when our ancestors dwelled amongst nature and wild animals. But everything changed with the advent of the modern world we live in now. What once was meant to help us survive has become a bane to everyone living in the demanding, modern times of today. It has become the scourge of our lives. Stress is not only a state of mind but it is also a dangerous syndrome that bears weight on our physical bodies. Chronic stress can be the cause for subtle changes in your body that can go unnoticed. Some of the more subtle but very dangerous effects of stress are its capability of killing the brain cells, and adding dangerous fat to the belly and waist area, exacerbating the likelihood of developing serious illnesses. Stress even has the power of unraveling our chromosomes. Stress is a lethal syndrome that can plague not only the body but the mind as well.

With over 3 decades of work and extensive, continued research on stress has allowed us to take a closer look at what stress truly is as it continues to reveal more. The decades long research on stress has given us further understanding of how stress impacts our body and our brain. Our social standing even has a great effect on whether or not we are more prone to stress. The toll that stress takes on in the body is astounding and great; it doesn't only affect the physical body but also the mind, playing off each other, making physical and mental conditions worse.

Adrenaline and glucocorticoids is the combination of hormones and backbone to the body's stress response. When these are turned on and set off for no apparent reason on an unending basis, is when stress begins to work against us. By not turning off the stress response when reacting to life's speed bumps we swim in a tub of destructive hormones. Even though the event we face is not a life or death situation, stress brings about physiological changes in us. We begin to hyperventilate, our muscles tense, our hearts hammer in our chest.

Ironically, the stress response becomes more damaging than the stressor itself because the stressors become physiological babble that we fall for and ultimately cause more destruction. The very same hormones that are meant to warn us of danger are the same ones that cause the silent trauma to our minds and bodies. Let's inspect the causes, symptoms and remedies for stress a bit more as we progress along.

Table of Contents

Chapter One: Stress: An Introduction

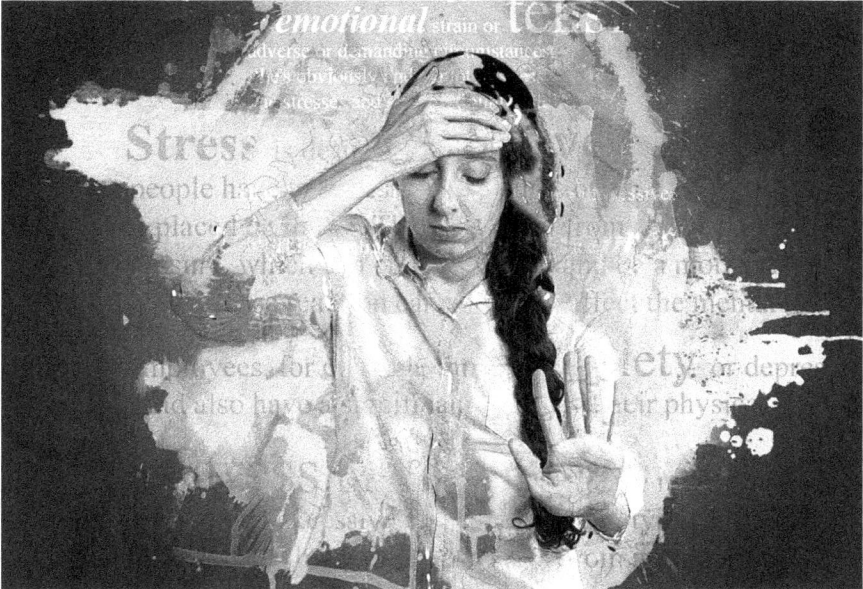

Stress - a word we hear all too frequently that oftentimes, it almost seem that it has lost its meaning in terms of what it truly is; the method of how our bodies and minds respond to a given situation or demand, dished out by random, unusual or everyday events, by means of dealing with what presents itself as a situation not typical of our routine. Almost all types of stipulations thrown at people can be considered stressors which play a part in a person's physical and mental shifts. Don't get us wrong. There are many forms of stress and not all of it is bad. Are you surprised?

Maybe you are and maybe you're not. But the point of us, being here, now is to shed more light on the matter, because stress is a reality we all have to live with, no matter how old we are, no matter what color skin we were born with, no matter our orientation, status or gender.

Possibly the first experience of stress we, as people, go through, is the day we are born and are introduced to the world outside of our mother's body. The process of being birthed takes a toll on us which suddenly alters our physical and mental state Compared to the warmth and safety of the womb, the world, upon our introduction to it is nothing like the secluded haven of our mother's belly.

We are handled and roused to life outside the secure sanctuary of our blissful, undisturbed, floating existence into a world of people calling out instructions and orders, passing us on from one person to another, inserting sucky tubes and poking us with needles (when required). It is an environment that is nothing at all similar to the almost quiet world we had existed in for the past 9 months. It is situations like these that we grow into as we mature and become more aware of expectations and the demands of our lives in general.

Stress, in its many forms and variations of encroachments, affects every one of us no matter what stage in our lives and since there is no cure to curb stress, our only real tool to manage it knows what stress is all about and what we can do to alleviate the physical and mental effects it has on us.

There were those who argued that if indeed stress comes about from a non-specific situation then the reaction should all be identical in individuals who experience similar stressors. But the longer research on stress went on and the more individuals put through experiment, the more it didn't seem right to come to any conclusive answers about type, origin or cause of stress. So further research was done which enlightened researchers to understand that various experimental studies done resulted in the revelation of the types of stressors that result in the release of stress hormones when one is under some sort of stress. These are varied in the responses and different for all of us with only some commonality in the specific situations which affect all of us.

Stress impacts us all in different ways and what sets stress effects off in each of us is just as unique as we are, although there are some generalizations of the causes of stress which we all usually identify with, like death and divorce there are other factors that trigger the release of stress us. Researchers over the course of time discovered that stress hormones reacted differently from one another; there are similar elements in situations that heighten the stress hormones of a person.

There are some, but not all, situations that can cause great anxiety and stress in a person. We'll be talking about more of the possible causes of stress in this compilation of useful information about these everyday syndromes. We shall delve into finding out how it not only affects the physiology of our body, but we shall also let you in on what you can do to manage the form of stress that may get in the way of our manner of everyday living.

Stress Hormones

The adrenal gland is where both adrenaline and glucocorticoids originate. It is located right above the kidney. The adrenal gland is what kicks off when an individual is faced with a high stress situation. Adrenaline is a neurotransmitter and hormone which is produced by the adrenal glands. It takes part in the sympathetic nervous system and sets off the acute stress response, commonly known as the fight or flight response when a person faces a high stress, exciting or dangerous situation. Glucocorticoids are a steroid hormone which also comes from the adrenal glands and works primarily as immunosuppressive and anti-inflammatory.

These hormones are essential to the fight and flight response in a highly stressful situation. When these are activated for an extended period of time with no particular physiological reason, our bodies, particularly the regulation of our organs, are disrupted. In a threatening, dangerous or exhilarating event, these hormones are temporary and a person recovers after the event. An example of a non-threatening activity is, going to an amusement park and getting on the wildest roller coaster ride. We would experience shortness of breath, a hammering of our hearts and a rush of blood. This example is one of fun, where after the event; our bodies slowly regulate and return to normal functioning.

When the adrenal gland reacts to a high-stress situation like this, we can safely say that our bodies are working for us in terms of providing the bodily responses required by us to "survive" a situation. This "survival" state changes drastically when the stress that is felt by a person is constant and unrelenting. When there is no call for both hormones to be active and they are, the body is in constant battle with the hormones. The absence of a reason for this response makes it dangerous for the person experiencing the usual reactions to a stressful or threatening situation.

In order to be free of stress you first have to understand what is causing the stress. Is it fact or thought? There are times when the cause of our stress is not factual but what we suppose a situation presents. If we are able to differentiate and isolate the situation, we would be able to better manage and handle the stressor. If we can learn to understand that stress begins in our minds by way of things we think about and suppose, we would come to understand that we can actually manage and control the stress that is plaguing us.

Let's cite a situation as an example. Take for example your job. You might think that it's a demanding one, and you think that it is too stressful for you. But then, take a look at the other people who have the same job as you do. Do they appear to not experience the same amount of stress that you do. How is that? When in fact both you and your colleague have the same job? It is most likely because what causes you stress are not the same stressor they experience.

Chapter Two: A Brief History of Stress

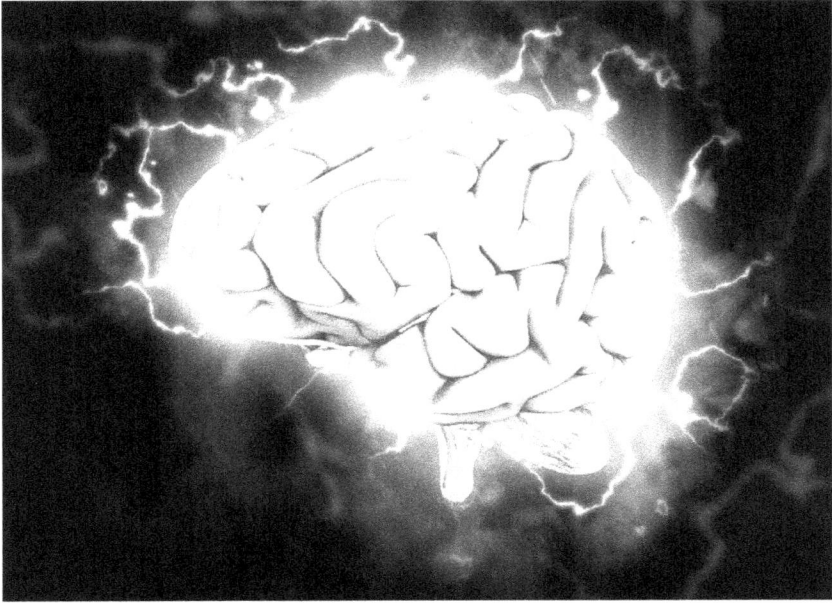

The origins of stress obviously came along with the emergence of man in the world but then stress was only recently given a name as great minds of science delved into the study of how it originates in different individuals. The term stress is a term borrowed from the arena of physics, by one of the minds who researched on stress, Hans Selye. The Hungarian born Selye chanced upon the notion of the G.A.S. or the General Adaptation Syndrome and later wrote about the condition in Nature, a British journal in the summer of 1936. The Hungarian doctor, who graduated top of his class, later earned his doctorate in organic chemistry.

As a young student of medicine, Hans Selye noticed that patients who suffered from various ailments and diseases would typically display similar symptom of "looking sick." Through years of observation and documentation of events relevant to his studies, Selye later described the symptoms, which he called the General Adaptation Syndrome; how the body responds to the demands it goes through.

It was later discovered that there were a host of other components that caused stress. But the groundbreaking findings of Selye had led to the further studies of the condition our bodies go through. However, many did not share the doctor's theory that stress comes about from a non-specific phenomenon. That is because there was present evidence of the onset of stress to one who has just lost a loved one, dealing with illness in the family, problems with work or finances, frustration, etc., also displayed to give effect to stress hormones elevating.

Let's take a look at the arguments and theories of Hans Selye's about General Adaptation Syndrome a little more and revisit the research of the multi-awarded doctor providing his evidence of stress impacting health.

Selye's General Adaptation Syndrome Theories

The doctor states that the first stage of G.A.S. is the initial reaction of a person to a given stressor and when one displays the "fight or flight" response. During this stage of the onset of a stressful situation, a human is zapped of the energy to supply to other systems of our body, like our immune system, thereby heightening the possibility of ailment in the person. The second stage, should the reaction progress to it, is when the body starts to get used to experiencing the stress by adapting to the situation, but the trouble with adaptation and resistance is how it affects the body's equilibrium because of where the stress concentrates on the body.

According to Dr. Selye, the final stage of a long span of exposure to stress breaking down the body's capability of warding off ailments because stress slowly reduces the ability of the person's immune system. Dr. Selye believed that patients who were exposed to long term stress could possibly develop a heart attack or be affiliated with a grave infection because of the lack of resistance of the body to ailments.

Decades after Dr. Selye's presentation of the G.A.S. theory, stress has been a field that many have studied and extensively researched. Perhaps it is because times and generations have shown not only the similarities of the elements of stress but also the diversity of other situations that brings about stress and the varied reactions of the people going through the experience. One stressor is not necessarily affecting all the same way and so ongoing discussions and discoveries made since then have truly furthered the initial theories of Dr. Hans Selye.

Chapter Three: Types of Stress and Stress Management

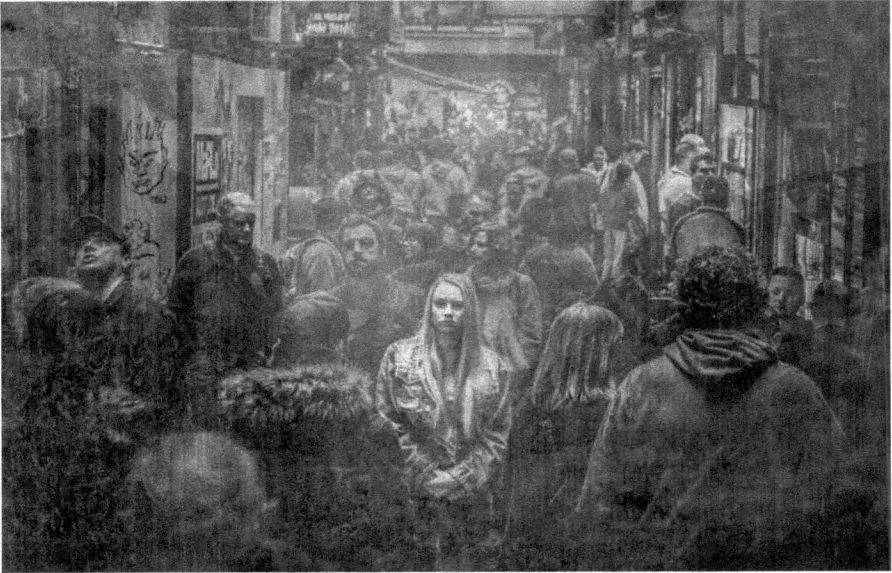

Stress serves us well in situations when our senses kick into alert to respond with quick reaction such as in situations where danger can pose threat to the safety of a person or the security of a loved one. Stress can in fact give us the ability to take calculated measures to preserve our existence and peace of mind. An experienced mountain climber, on a challenging climb, can make use of the stress hormones released to work toward their favor. The stress brought about the excitement or anxiety of new trails as they climb gives them the ability to employ skills that will keep them safe as they ascend the mountain.

They are prepared and have a general idea of what to expect during the trek and are experienced enough to understand that there things to watch out for throughout the expedition. On the other hand, an inexperienced individual, if they we to be challenged go up the same mountain by way of the same trek as the experienced ones, the latter will display a more alarming spike in the release of stress hormones. Increased levels of stress hormones released could not only affect the physical balance (labored breathing, constricted muscles, strained bowels) could disorient the novice "hiker" leading them to make uncalculated deductions that could be detrimental to their survival.

Stress can be categorized in groups and we shall talk about these categories separately as we provide some examples which may help lead the reader to understanding the gravity of each sort of stress as well as some situations which may trigger stress.

Chronic Stress

Chronic Stress can be detrimental to the health of an individual. It contributes to a host of grave illnesses that are chronic, severe or life-threatening. This is experienced by an individual or individuals for a lasting period of time which develops to the more severe kind of stress.

This is the kind of stress experienced which is constant. Some examples could be helplessness through poverty. The inability to provide for the family is one very stressful situation indeed and can cause all sorts of dysfunction to the patient which could cause them to suffer from stress.

Another reason for chronic stress is the presence of numerous problems within the family. Coming from a dysfunctional family makes people step up in ways that sets off their fight or flight instincts and if not managed in a way that is effective for the individual, can develop all sorts of bad situation responses by the patient suffering stress in this environment.

It is not unusual to hear about family members of all ages showing symptoms of stress because of the unconventionally challenging lifestyles each of the family member lives on a daily basis. Couples suffering marital problems are candidates for stress. During stages of marital discord, couples have been found to have different reactions and had varied measures of stress levels in response to the same demand.

Being unhappy in one's job, whether it is a bad paying one or employment that goes against your beliefs or morals, is another source of mental anguish that is caused by and exacerbated by stress. Heart and lung diseases as well as some cancers are attributed to long term stress.

Episodic Acute Stress

Individuals who have episodic acute stress are people who seem to be in constant crisis mode. They are individuals who express strong reactions to what they would perceive as a negative situation and respond in an equally negative manner. They are the ones who are irritable at the slightest provocation, short-tempered and typically on the edge. They are the ones who worry about things that are possible and imagined. They usually have a bleak outlook about things and feel helpless. The problem with those with episodic acute stress is that this is usually because they have come to accept a sort of defeat about stress being a part of life.

Acute Stress

Acute stress is another form of stress that is not as bad as it sounds. Acute stress is basically the common responses of our bodies and minds to a demanding situation. It can be as unusual and accidental like a near miss, road incident. It can also be a response to the defense mechanisms of the body when in an argument with family member. It can be the physical and mental reactions your body reacts to on the micro level when undergoing some sort of employment pressure.

Severe cases of acute stress can stem from traumatic experiences, like if a person becomes a victim of sexual abuse. a violent crime or traumatic experience. People, who develop acute stress suddenly because of a sudden and very unpleasant experience, can lead for the person to suffer mental health issues, like depression and PTSD. On a more positive note, isolated episodes of stress allow for the body and brain to learn from the situation, making the individual better able to make better future decisions.

Chapter Four: Common Modern Day Stressors

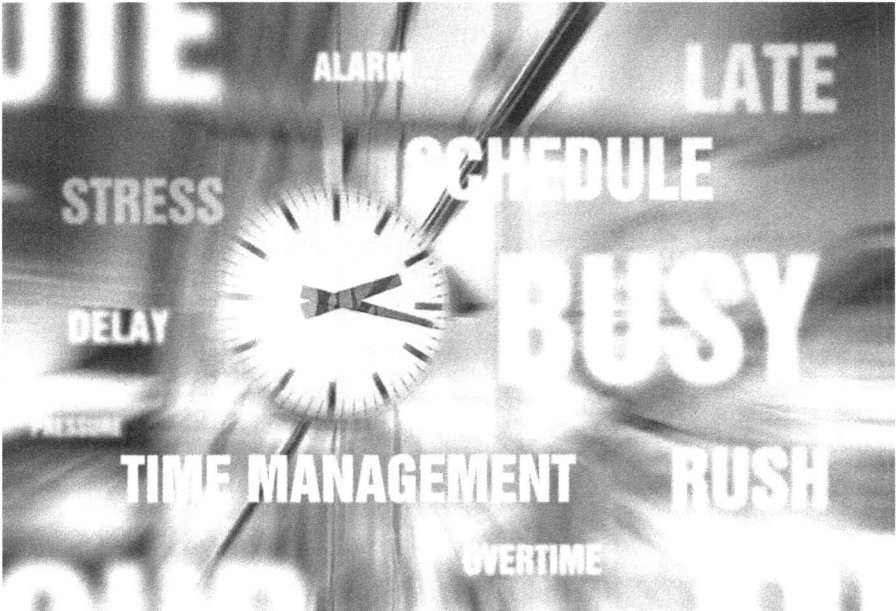

All of us deals with stress differently, and stressors are different for each one of us. One stressor is not necessarily what the stressors would be for another. In most cases, identifying what elicits the stress in us can be pretty straightforward and obvious. Stress can stem from a bad relationship, an argument with someone, subpar working or living conditions, and suffering from health issues are just some of the more obvious reasons for the onset of stress. In other cases, determining the root cause of the stress being experienced is more difficult.

Finding the origin of your anxiety can be a little more challenging especially if the stress does not manifest itself in forms we recognize and understand. If you find yourself feeling more stressed out than usual try keeping a journal of what sets off the stress hormones in you. This is a good way of recording what it is that causes you uninvited stress and worry.

When you start to feel these emotions and physical reactions overwhelm you, it is a good time to take stock f the situation and answer questions like the following:

- Is it someone in particular that sets off the stress alarms in me?
- Is it a particular place that triggers dark emotions?
- What time of the day do I feel most on edge?
- Do I make unsound decisions under stress?

When we start recognizing the patterns, this will be when we would be better able to understand what triggers stress for us. When we are able to understand these, then we shall be better equipped to handle the stress.

Some of the things that we worry about is what stresses us out on a daily basis. These could be mundane things and others are more pressing matters that either needs our attention or situations that bring about anxiety that we have no control over. Research has shown that an average person would suffer between two hours and thirty minutes stressing out about things such as, where to have lunch, and what to have for lunch. We worry about how we look and what to wear. We worry if there is enough gas in the car. We fret over payments we need to make and if there is enough food in the refrigerator.

These concerns are just some of the more common causes of stress that we can identify. For those who work, some of their more stressful concerns include job satisfaction, workplace environment, and keeping balance between home and work life. More and more, keeping a work-life balance has become very important to working individuals. Not surprisingly, working people are very concerned about how they are managing and balancing their daily lives, including family, career, and self.

Stress is sometimes higher for some people, especially those who have families. We shall be talking about the more common stressors that most of us experience on a daily basis and look into what we can do to alleviate some of the effects of stress when it rears its head.

It has been noted that all of our minor worries cost us at least two hours and 28 minutes of our lives stressing, every day. Women's teams to stress out more than men do with women spending at least 2 hours and 35 minutes each day on worries and men spending a little less than that at 2 hours and 18 minutes each day on the average. This data shows us that yes indeed women do worry more than men do but with the very slight difference in time spent worrying women and men are not so different after all. It has been noted that stress levels usually peak at the beginning of the week on a Monday morning, sometime before lunch, when people usually spend time planning out the hectic schedule of the week ahead.

Research over the decades has revealed that although the kind of stressors which set off the release of stress hormones are varied with each individual, there are is in fact a commonality in the elements to the situation which causes the stress hormones of people experiencing stress to rise. These studies showed that the novelty of a situation especially unexpected and unanticipated, was one of the reasons for stress hormones to elevate. Another situation that would cause stress hormones to increase is the sense of losing control over a situation as well as when there is a perceived threat to the person or their ego.

Top 10 moments which lead tutorial stress levels in women. 56% of women are said to stress out during a job interview as opposed to 47% of men. 44% women worry about not earning enough, whereas 33% males stress about the amount of money they make.

At 43% there are more women who are worried about getting a presentation or a speech in front of a crowd then 37% of the male population. 41% more women worry about the lack of time during the day as opposed to 26% of males who feel they do not have enough time in a day to do what they need to do. Women, at 40%, worry more about their first day on the job than men (29%) do. Men worry less about being cheated on pegging the numbers at 17%, than women do at 32%. Women, at 34%, stress over disagreements with friends, whereas men are more cavalier about it at 23%. Men worry more about job security at 27%, whereas women, at 24%, seem a little more secure about their paycheck source.

Both men and women worry about being underachievers, almost equally, with women pegged at 24% and men at 23%. Women seem to worry more about being first time parents, making them either prepare for an eventual arrival of their addition, or position women in a manner where they can get all the help they need or afford. Some of the other things that men worry about are going on first dates, concerned about not having enough time and losing hair.

The national mental health institute says that 40 million adults in the USA are affected by anxiety, with countless more who suffer from depression related disorders. It has been reported that about 18% of adults suffer from depression related conditions while the rest of us are particularly stressed out during child-rearing ages and prime productivity between the ages of 18 to 55. However there are some folks who, for specific reasons, suffer more from stress and anxiety for various reasons that could be due to a genetic mutation or their strong stressful experiences could be triggered by episodes caused by past trauma.

A person who seems less equipped to deal with the pressure of stressful events could be suffering from an underlying, undiagnosed medical condition of the brain. The stress could also be attributed to an idiosyncratic chemical imbalance. Often times we witness similar situations experienced by different individuals that result to totally different outcomes. Some people who have been able to have themselves diagnosed for disorders suffer more intense versions of the same situation than other people do because they are more affected by circumstance of the situation which they feel they have no control over.

The life man lives presently is quite different from how early man lived on a daily basis. The challenges are certainly incomparable in terms of how ancient man's days went as to how our present lives play out. The modern world is riddled with people suffering from anxiety and depression than those of our distant ancestors because we are forced, by modern times, to interact with a more diverse group of people. We come across new people more now than our ancient counterparts did. And because of the growing population of the world collectively, as well as the mix of race, age, religion, morals, and beliefs, we are confronted with diversity in terms of knowledge, skills and values.

Religious beliefs, the politics we subscribe to, and the music we enjoy, are just some of the obvious differences we share as human beings. Figuring out the best way to get along with people is a matter that most of us worried about. There is a delicate balance between standing up for your own beliefs while respecting another person's values without compromising yours. It will seem that we are always on the edge in terms of avoiding confrontation or disagreement. In other words, the question about whether our brains are well equipped to deal with the vast degree of diversity we are faced with on a daily basis.

Chapter Five: Symptoms and Effects of Stress

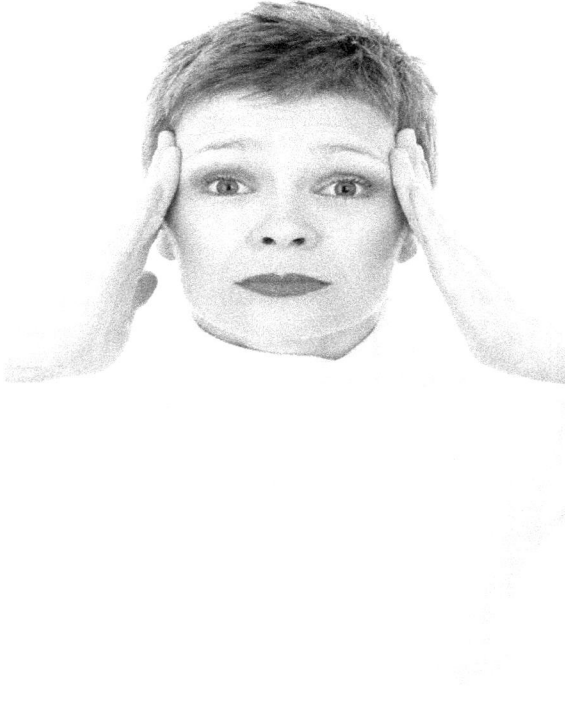

Stress isn't all bad and in fact in tiny doses some types of stress can actually motivate us to work better, even smarter, when under pressure. Now, operating under pressure for an extended length of time will indeed start taking a toll on the body and mind if left unchecked. Under these conditions the individual begins to operate from the 2nd stage of stress which is forming a sort of adaptation to the given situation.

As we deal with any given stressful situation on this level, we begin to show signs of our physical bodies taking on more and more of the stance of resistance. Needless to say, this is when the condition starts to become troublesome. When your body kicks into high gear and you find yourself typically on edge and overwhelmed, it is time to take care of yourself and step back to realign your equilibrium.

The important thing right now is to take back what you can by informing yourself of what it is that you are facing. By naming the condition, you have just given yourself the chance to start on a path that will help you get through stressful situations by way of learning to recognize the symptoms of chronic, or recurring, stress. This recognition, allows us to take measures to lessen the side effects of stress, in some cases, through some techniques one can apply.

The Positive and Negative Effects of Stress

Stress is the way your body is signaled on how to survive any given situation which is out of the ordinary of your routine experiences. Stress physically signals your body to respond to some kind of internal or external demand or threat which swiftly puts us in heightened senses alert, no matter if the situation is imagined or real. This is called the fight or flight response, and it is the initial stage of a series of stages when responding to stress. In a way, stress is your body's way of protecting you by helping us to stay focused and alert. A good example would be stress under a medical emergency; under this kind of demanding events, one can help them by staying focused and getting the help they need. Or to react in a fashion that would put them out of a dire situation like an accident. Stress can in fact, in certain situations help us, recognize a threat and react accordingly.

Stress is what actually brings you through a presentation, keeping you on your toes. It allows you to meet expectations put upon your shoulders by helping sharpen concentration. It is what helps you focus when studying for a big exam. However, there is a limit to everything and when all of these start compiling and starts to become overwhelming for the individual this is when stress becomes detrimental to our health.

Stress not only affects the body in manners like shortness of breath, quickened pulse and heartbeat. The release of stress hormones, like cortisol and adrenaline, sets your physical body on emergency mode ass your blood pressure rises, your muscles tighten and your senses are on high alert. All these in work together heightens our energy and strength, speeding up our reaction, in preparation for a response.

Operating on this level on a prolonged period of time can begin affecting the normal functional balance of our body, which may lead to more serious medical conditions. In other ways, prolonged stress can alter the mood of a person, it can affect ones productivity and take a general toll on the person's quality of life.

The nervous system, for all the wonderful work it does for us, is not able to recognize the difference between physical and emotional threats. When a person is faced with a stressful situation such as facing a work deadline, or burdened with a mountain of bills to pay, our bodies go on overdrive and react as if we were facing a life threatening situation.

When your body is always primed on react on red alert, it can be difficult to take hold of the situation to regulate the physiology of the body. It also interrupts with our ability to decide what to do or act too strongly to a situation. It is like a cycle which needs to be recognized in order to distinguish what skills to employ in order to deal accordingly so as not to encourage the onset of more serious conditions. Chronic stress can commonly lead to more serious health issues if it disrupts your body equilibrium often enough.

Stress suppresses the immune system of a person whilst disrupting the digestive as well as the reproductive system of an individual.

A person who experiences chronic stress has a higher likelihood of developing more serious diseases and are at higher risk for stroke and heart attack. Stress can induce speed up the aging process of a person caught under the pressures of stress. Not only does it display itself in terms of outward, physical appearances, in form of perhaps wrinkles or dark rings under the eyes, stress can in fact trigger off more serious conditions because your organs and systems of a person who undergo chronic stress are on perpetual overdrive.

Fight, Flight or Freeze Response

Fear is an important aspect of our survival and our bodies do something really remarkable when we undergo any form of stress. Our bodies begin to react to a threat before we are even aware of what the threat might be; when we are faced with danger even a millisecond count. At the first brightening of danger early warning signals are sent to the brain via the optic nerve into a tiny and primitive brain center called the amygdala.

This prepares our body for action. The next thing that happens in a threatening situation is that nerve pulses are set off down the spine to the adrenal glands near our kidneys. When this happens our body releases adrenaline hormones putting us on heightened alert. Adrenaline is a hormone that can overcome her body in a split second. As adrenaline reaches our lungs we find ourselves breathing faster and taking more oxygen in general and also make your heart beat faster.

Oxygen rich blood is then distributed to our muscles charging them for action waiting for the signal to run from apparent and possible danger OR stand your ground and fight. All this happens even before our conscious mind realizes, understands and registers a threat. This reaction to fear has evolved over millions of years known as the fight or flight response.

When your amygdala is hijacked by stress it responds to an emotional threat. And the potential emotional attack or threat brings on the fight or flight response. When we are in a non-life threatening situation, when it is a supposed threat to our emotions and ego and our amygdala kicks in, our bodies react just as it would in a dangerous situation. When this happens the amygdala takes over the neocortex part of the brain. This is the rational and thinking area of our brain.

When the amygdala hijacks the neocortex we are robbed of the proper faculties to think straight and reason logically. Mediate response is a malfunction of the ability to recall or to remember some details. When this happen recovery time from a situation as such takes about 3 to 4 hours to be reset to its proper function. This scenario is repeated time again if not recognized for what it is will become a vicious cycle of adaptation to the stress.

In order to hijack the amygdala from hijacking the new cortex it is up to us to be able to identify what the stressor is. Name the trigger or in motion this keeps the neocortex engaged and active as it helps you prevent the amygdala from taking over. Call it out, give the emotion and situation a name. Recognize it for what it is.

Keep the neocortex engaged by being present at the moment and breathing. By breathing we get the oxygen back into the neocortex, bypassing the signals sent by the amygdala. The amygdala basically shuts everything down. Allowing the amygdala to take control over your responses negates the functionality of the new cortex when in fact you want to keep the functionality of the neocortex in top shape during a stressful situation. It is the new cortex that gives you the ability to figure out solutions not just one but multiple solutions to a situation.

The amygdala prevents that from happening once it is allowed to hijack your neocortex. Many people were under stress when face in a situation that is not regular routine would usually want to flee from the situation. Other people would stand her ground and fight. These are logical solutions to a situation where you find your life the life of your loved ones to be under mortal danger.

The problem is these are also the reactions and responses of our brain and body to a non-life threatening situation. And what are these non-life-threatening situations that plague us on a daily basis on a weekly basis on a monthly basis? That would be work responsibilities, bills to pay, family to provide for, putting food on the table, mortgage payments, car payments, acceptance in society, etc. all these are basically things that you cannot run away from nor can you fight them.

If your amygdala kicks in and overpowers your neo cortex, it basically prevents us from finding out the best solution to the problem. What happens if it freezes as immobilizes us preventing us from making ways to fulfill a payment, a responsibility or a task. This is the time when you will need the full functionality of your neocortex to be able to find ways discover solutions and make preparations. This is the time when you will need to relax breathe then we doubt do it again and think I way of your neocortex.

Is it a time when the rationality of your new cortex will serve you well in this seemingly stressful situation you find yourself in. We need to be able to use the full functionality of our rational brain and not allow the irrationality of the signals sent by the amygdala because once the amygdala takes over the new cortex logical thinking clear ideas and rational thought is thrown out the window leaving us a heaped pile of stressed mess.

Another way to manage stress is to think positively, to appreciate the good in your life. There are many ways for you to be able to appreciate now. Stepping away from the stressor for a minute to relieve yourself of the pressure is one manner of getting your head on straight. If you have a furry pet, take a minute or two and spend some time cuddling with your pet (pets are said to have an ability of releasing tension from the body and mind) and then go back to the situation at hand; you just might find that a solution or at the very least, relief, is obtained.

When our minds are supplied with the proper amount of oxygen, we are better able to think clearly. Or perhaps, you find solace in music. Take time off and listen to an inspiringly upbeat song or two before you tackle what needs your attention. You may not get instant solutions but your head is clear and able to, with possible solutions which you can later apply toward the stress factor.

Symptoms of Stress

Even though we don't often realize it, stress affects our health in ways that are detrimental and frustrating. Stress has a way of masking itself through sleeplessness and chronic headaches. Stress zaps us of energy and strength that it affects our productivity. Stress is sneaky because it not only contributes to the deterioration of our health, but also is the culprit for the mood and behavioral changes in us. Like a thief in the night that can catch one unawares at any given time, so can stress jump out at you for a variety of reasons, when unexpected.

The problem and danger of this is that a person who experiences stress often enough has pretty much "learned" to adapt their physiology to the stress they undergo during trigger events that it begins to seem the norm. When this stage is where a person operates from, stress begins to take a toll on the individual's health.

For many, since they are not aware of the amount of energy our bodies spend to handle stress, start displaying signs and symptoms of overload. For one, people under unrelenting, extended stress, may employ poor judgment, when once they did not. They have a harder time concentrating on things that need their attention and this can be coupled with constantly entertaining worrying thoughts. A person who under stress can feel panicked with negativity, sometimes gripping them with the inability to do anything (part of the fight, flight or freeze response people go through when under distress. And because they are consumed by anxiety, a person under stress can begin showing signs of memory problems. A person experiencing stress experiences physical and mental effects like:

- Sleep problems
- Anxiety
- Headache
- Restlessness
- Stomach upset
- Lack of focus or motivation
- Muscle tension or pain
- Feelings that overwhelm
- Change in sex drive
- Anger and irritability
- Chest pain
- Fatigue
- Depression and sadness
- Angry outbursts
- Smoking
- Little physical activity or exercise

- Undereating
- Overeating
- Abuse of alcohol
- Abuse of drugs
- Social withdrawal

The problem with stress is that it silently creeps up on us, and catches us unaware. The manner our physical bodies respond to the demands of any given situation that one may find stressful is the danger of not recognizing the origin of the ailment. Chronic stress tilts the axis of the body's equilibrium and affects not only our physical health but our mental stability as well.

Stress can bring about the onset of autoimmune diseases - diseases where your own body attacks its own self. Some examples of autoimmune diseases are type 1 diabetes, rheumatoid arthritis, multiple sclerosis, Systemic Lupus Erythematosus (SLE), Sjogren's syndrome, psoriasis, scleroderma, Cushing's disease, alopecia, Addison's disease, Polycystic Ovary Syndrome (PCOS), Inflammatory Bowel Syndrome (IBD), Ulcerative Colitis, and Crohn's disease just to name a few. In fact there are between 80 to 100 autoimmune diseases that can affect people.

Chapter Six: Dealing and Managing Stress

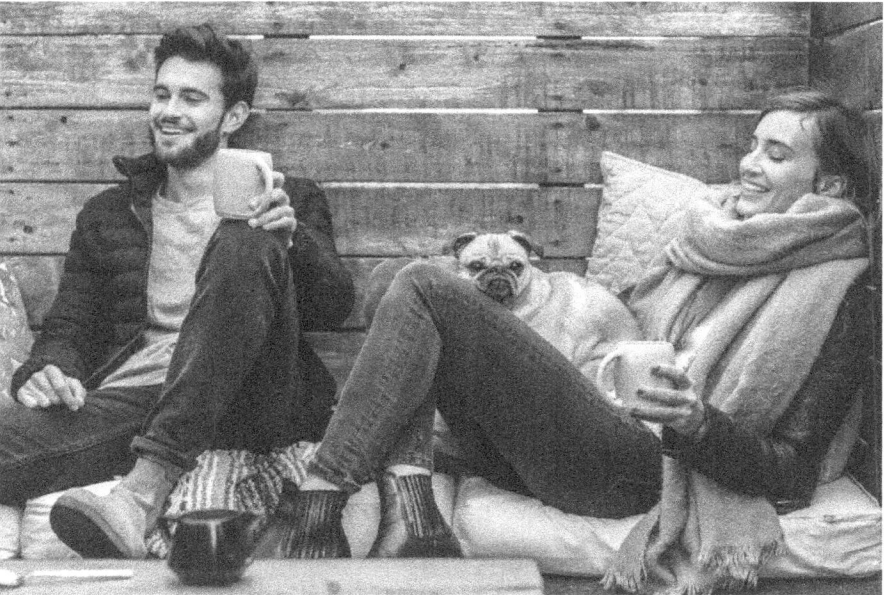

Stress, like opinion, is subjective and relative to the person experiencing the situation that leads to triggering stress responses. And that is how stress affects us. It sets off a series of physical responses which aims to compensate, and or protect us. Stress is what causes chemicals and hormones to be produced by your body in order to aid you to face the music and rise up to the challenge, so to speak. Is there a cure for stress? Short answer is, knowing what stresses you and learning how to handle any particular stressful situation in a manner that is non-destructive.

It is after all a situation that can affect not only your physical health but your mental health as well. Long answer is, the basic understanding of stress and how it affects you, somehow allows you to take back the reins and give you the privilege of steering yourself out of the situation causing you stress.

Controlled studies and informal suppositions of people under stress showed that not all stress factors are the same for all. Under controlled circumstances, individuals who were exposed to varied situations showed varied results in terms of what gives stress to an individual. A lot of people think of stress as an event that occurs to them, be it a form of possible harm or, on the other end of the spectrum, encouragement. Then there are those who suppose that stress is how our bodies, our minds and behavior respond when something stressful happens.

When an event which raises stress hormones our immediate response is to, first, mentally evaluate the situation, thereby allowing us to deduce if the situation poses danger to us, once we have assessed the situation, we decide how to deal with it. When we are confident that we have the skills to deal with a particular situation, this is not deemed as a stress factor. However, this changes radically when we are in an unusual situation that makes us realize that the demands of the situation is no match for our skill to overpower.

There are circumstances in life which prove to be stress-provoking, but in the end it's our perception of whether we are equipped with the abilities to handle the situation or not. It is how we perceive the stress-provoking incident and how we react to the stress factor which determines the impact of the situation on our overall health. Understanding oneself and knowing the strengths and weaknesses one has, they would be able to learn how they can handle difficult situations better.

How to Deal and Manage Stress

A support group who rallies behind you, no matter what, is another stress reducing factor. When you have family or friends who make themselves available to you, you are less likely to wallow in stress for too long. This would be a good time to identify the people in your life that you are sure you can count on in times of trouble laying stress. They may not necessarily have the solution to your problem, they may not know what to say to you during your time of distress but the important factor in all of this is that you have people in your life who how empathy and who listen.

The next time you feel that you are being hijacked by the amygdala sit down and write about all the feelings that you are encountering at the moment. Identify them, give it a name, and word it out. You don't necessarily need to solve it at the very moment, just write down a situation that set off your stress hormones and list all the emotions that feel. Be specific as you can be.

Once you have done that and when you are later on feeling much stronger, come back and address every one of those emotions that you had listed down. Revisit the concerns you wrote when you have confidently recovered from the highjack and figure out if what you had listed, all of them whether they be valid concerns or irrational ideas and thoughts. Writing down a list allows you to understand the origin of the stress factor thereby allowing you to make better, more rational decisions later when your neocortex is hijacked by your amygdala. Now this may not be the solution to your problem next time but it will reveal a pattern of how your rational brain is being overtaken by the irrational part of your head.

Make this a habit. Make it a point that every time you are in the grips of a stressful situation that you write down the root cause of the stress. You want to put down on paper how the situation makes you feel. Write everything down no matter how silly think it may sound put it down on paper.

When you revisit it later on then you can figure out what is this a good response to that stress factor that set off all my stress hormones to go haywire. Being able to answer each and every one of those feelings will validate whether or not it was something that deserved to be stressed over. Most of the time you would realize that the stress you had felt at the onset of the stress factor did not match the intensity of your reaction.

Chapter Seven: Stress Prevention and Management of Stress – Related Illnesses

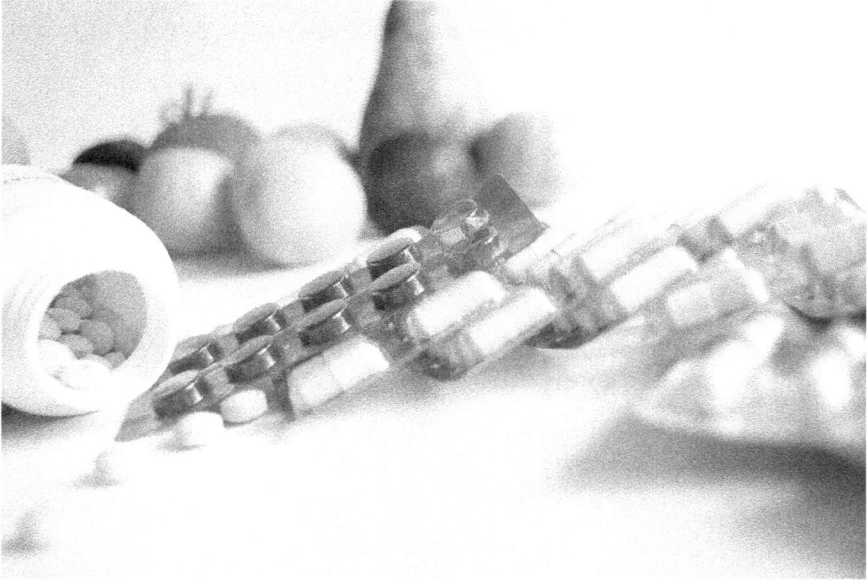

Each person deals with stress in their own way. And this is not to say that these are voluntary reactions but these are involuntary responses our bodies make in order to compensate for the effects of the causes of factors of the stress. Our bodies respond to the effects of stress differently. Some people may experience shortness of breath, and exhibit trembling and tremors. Others may exhibit stress physically, getting stomach aches, headaches or they may get sick frequently. It is impossible to eliminate stress completely, given the demands life, society, our jobs, our relationships, and of course, our own selves, impose upon us.

With stress being a part of most societies, with a set of different commonalities and variances, making it a point to identify individual and specific stressors, can allow the individual to take back some of the control by employing stress management techniques to lessen the stress effects on one's overall health. Knowing what demands the most of your energy, identifying what depletes you of the energies your body needs to function optimally, is one manner on how you can overcome the negativity brought about by those situations. Read about some of the ways one can help cope with stress below.

- Taking care of your health is vital to not only your physical health but your mental stability as well. Taking care of your health means that you will need to be mindful about what you eat. Sticking to a balanced diet feeding not only the body but beneficial as well to mental balance is a healthy step toward combating stressful situations. When an individual exercises regularly even if it just a quick, 30-minute brisk walk around the block, or a regular bike ride to work, getting the proper, and moderate workout for your health is essential to curbing the effects of stress. Having the proper amount of sleep at the correct time is a catalyst for a clear head. A good night's rest allows for better decision making.

- Sometimes, a good ear is all you need to blow off some steam and avoid further stress from progressing and worsening. Support is usually found from friends and or family by talking about the source of the demands on your person. It is easy to isolate oneself under stressful situations or when going through a difficult spell - avoid staying away from being around company which may lead to more serious mental issues like depression and suicide.

- Learn to remove yourself from the stressful situation. Sometimes, stepping away from the situation which causes you stress can in fact help you clear your head of the cause of your anxiety. Taking the high road can also mean turning away from the situation that causes you stress. It is also good to be reminded that using drugs and alcohol as means of escaping the realities of a stressful event may help on a short term basis but can actually cause bigger and worse problems in the long run. The ill-effects of the use of illegal drugs, self-medication and excessive alcohol consumption during stressful events in one's life leads to dependency to substances that first does not help us in facing the situation, thereby learning how to make decisions on future responses.

Every person is bound to deal with stress on way or another simply because stress is part of like. What we need to keep in mind is that not all stress is bad because it does give us the ability to assess a situation and make calculated deductions about the best response to any given situation. Concern does creep in when stress is prolonged because of the impact it has on our overall health.

With most than a host of stressful situations waiting around the bend with each day we traverse, it is more than ever important to accept the stressors that can trigger off stress hormones. From minor everyday incidents that come along with the birth of each day to the more long-lasting, more chronic forms of stress that is put in the backburner of our everyday lives, tucked away and not dealt with by us. Proactively finding ways for you to be able to deal with the underlying, tucked away stressors in your life will empower you to better deal with the everyday challenges. To manage stress means to maintain a fulfilling and healthy life.

If we could see that there are thoughts are creating more stress and not our situation we would be better able to manage stress. Being able to recognize this is good news to you because then you would be equipped with the right skill set to recognize fact from supposed thoughts in your current situation. Keep in mind that you don't have to change your situation to be stressed free you just have to change the way you think about the situation.

In order to be free of what is creating the stress, we first need to identify what specific thoughts, stories or beliefs the stress originates from and to do this whenever you feel stressed ask yourself an honest question what outcome am I afraid of?

For example let's say you have a report that you need to submit to your boss and you worry about whether the report is accurate good enough and acceptable to your boss or perhaps you might be going out on a date you and you might be worried that the person you are going out with will not like you or perhaps you are preparing for an exam and you are worried that you might fail this test.

The next question to ask yourself after you've determined to answer for the first is what outcome I think is the best. Your answers maybe it would be best if I prepare the report we had of time and check that everything is in order for perhaps for your date you might say I'll just be myself and see where it goes from there and for exam you might give yourself an answer like "I need to learn to study more efficiently." When you determine the best outcome, you basically set yourself up to succeed. How, you may ask is this? Well, asking yourself about what is the best outcome, allow you to better prepare yourself. You are essentially avoiding the worst possible outcome to be free from your thoughts in order to be free from that specific stress.

Once you understand that your thoughts are creating your stress and want to identify the specific stress and next thing you have to do is to not believe that thought. This sounds like a radical and quite a difficult step to managing the stress but it is your way of helping yourself to illuminate unnecessary unmerited stressful thoughts.

When a person believes words to be true there is a corresponding emotion that goes along with the words you hear or think. Notice that, on the other hand, when you don't believe that there's any truth to the words you hear, no emotions are involved. Asking these questions and give a real honest answers from yourself enables you to identify what it is that is causing your stress.

When you have been able to honestly answer these questions then you have basically set yourself up to understand what it is you can do. Perhaps it's just a matter of being more prepared for a job interview it could also equate to you studying harder for an exam. You thereby eliminate the supposed thoughts that causes you stress. Stress and anxiety are only created by what you know. Stress cannot be created when you know that you are free. Uncertainty does not create stress but the nagging thoughts of supposition.

Once you realize that you don't know which outcome is better or worse, once you understand that uncertainty is a given, you allow yourself to be free of the stress and anxiety paving the way for you to do what is rightful. Knowing that uncertainty is evident, gives you the tools to prepare and look inward. Realizing that uncertainty will always be present gives us the opportunity to put the best versions of ourselves into action.

If you come to realize that the idea that good or bad could happen given a particular scenario (and be inventive with the scenarios) and give logical answers to these supposed bad outcomes, you will be able to understand that there are actually so many possible outcomes.

Take for example a person who feels unrecognized by their boss. One person may not find your worth in what you do, but there are other people who find you to be indispensable. Take a bad break up. Say you got really hurt from a bad split but this separation paved the way for perhaps a new and more fulfilling relationship with another person or maybe you discover that you are presently better off without the taxing relationship that ended. In other words, mindset is vital to managing stress.

We have been "programmed" by the demands of society to work under stressful conditions. Preparing for a test, a job interview, submitting a report, are just some of the realities we all experience. We don't know any other way of operating unless it's under circumstances of pressure and demand. Operating under pressure and fear (of rejection or reprimand) as the way to getting approval or success has been the norm for many of us.

When you are stressed while doing something, there is no fun or pleasure in the task at hand. You may procrastinate and put it off 'til the last minute because it does not give you the uplift of doing something you enjoy. Procrastinating only heightens the stress factor because, now, you're on limited time. On the other hand, if what you were doing gave you pleasure, if you enjoy what you do, you spend more time on this task, and it wouldn't bother you one bit. You look forward to doing it, and you carry out the task the best way possible because there is no accompanying stress to what needs to be done.

It is easier to be focused and creative when we are free from stress and anxiety. When we are free from stress, we are able to be more comfortable and authentic. Identify the source of the stress. Eliminate stressors by asking yourself logical questions about the root of the stress factor, and answer them just as honestly.

Stress makes us unhappy. It prevents us from being accessible to people. We are not pleasant to be around and this is manifested through the way we interact with others. So this is another vicious cycle in which we are trapped by the grips of stress. How, you may ask? Through isolation; when we are not pleasant to be around, our response (under stress) is to withdraw. We isolate ourselves from the company of others, thereby giving more way to the stress of insecurity. This becomes a lonely cycle unless we recognize and break the cycle! When you are not stressed and happy, you are better primed to help you get what you want.

Managing Other Health Conditions by Managing Stress

Other stress related health problems include dealing with emotional and mental conditions such as depression and anxiety. When a person goes under emotional stress, it can go either way with the individual becoming hyper social or as in others, would completely withdraw and remove themselves from any social interaction. Either way, most people who experience either one of these social phenomena, reports that it becomes very lonely.

A person who is under constant stress is pretty much always on the defensive, a person operating under this condition for a prolonged period of time without respite can begin showing signs of mood swings and behavioral changes. People under the constant strain of challenging situations could have unknowingly "modified" their systems to adapt to the hyper-drive they have gotten used to, putting further strain on an already frayed health system.

Apart from the aforementioned diseases, other medical conditions that can come about because of stress would be digestive illnesses. When a person is under stress, they often describe sensations in the pit of their stomachs that make it feel as if their guts are being ripped out or they describe a sinking sensation.

When stress activates the fight or flight response the nervous system shuts down the blood flow to the body's digestive system. Stress affects how your stomach muscles contract. It also decreases its ability to digest because of the lack of secretions needed to do so. Long term, chronic stress can cause some people's gastrointestinal system to become inflamed making them more susceptible to infection.

When a person is under stress, the esophagus goes into spasms and stress causes the increase of acid production in the stomach. The colon is affected by stress and can affect the person under stress to have diarrhea or bouts of constipation. When a person is under severe stress they could experience severe nausea. Although not the direct cause of conditions such as celiac disease, stomach ulcers or inflammatory bowel diseases, stress can in fact worsen these medical conditions.

What You Can Do

The conditions of where an individual lives and works are absolutely vital to health. One antidote to stress is perhaps seeking out a place where we have some sort of control. Much like removing oneself from a stressful situation, choosing how we can lower the instances of stress, whether routine, chronic or acute, is of vital importance to the body and mind of a human being.

When in doubt if it is indeed stress that is causing your illness, take action and get in touch with your physician to get a full check up to identify the cause of your malaise. Make sure that you get the proper amount of sleep and maintain a balanced diet. Sleep is important for all of us, not having enough sleep can cause us to become clouded, and irritable. Improper diet equates to not getting the proper nutrients one would need in order to supply the various parts of our bodies. Help yourself by avoiding alcohol and illicit substances. As tempting as the temporary relief they bring, the damage will be worse in the long run. Make it a point that you see your physician to check for other potential causes of the physical changes in you.

Resorting to surfing the Internet, watching television or playing video games may seem like good ways to get your mind off the stress hounding you, but these measures may in fact be more detrimental in the long run, increasing stress even more instead of decreasing it. A person suffering from the syndrome needs to proactively search for methods to manage stress. To say that one to relax and stay active is easy, it's a whole different ball game searching for ways to help oneself.

Have you ever done or said anything at the heat of the moment that you later regretted? Are you allowed your temper to get the best of you perhaps during rush hour or maybe you snapped irritability at a family member or a friend. Well it would be safe to say that most every one of us has been in this situation. This is your classic case of an amygdala hijack. The good news is you can actually train your brain to end the cycle of your amygdala over powering the neocortex through mindfulness to decrease the instances of reacting with your emotions.

The amygdala is the part of our brain that is responsible for emotional reactions, what we don't know is that this part of our brain is also a bit of a thief when activated because it has the power to overpower the neocortex, the part of our logical, rational brain, which is also responsible for sensory perception.

In essence a logical brain is over written by a surge of emotions. Commendation stressors activate the part of the brain that makes you want to fight or flee. Distressed or could be as simple as a text message is stuck in traffic not having dinner on time or a botched up meeting. All these stressors activate the inherited instinct we got from our prehistoric ancestors.

Knowing this we are no better able to identify the more common stressors of everyday life that sets off the reaction of the amygdala. It allows us to be more mindful about utilizing the functionality of our rational brain to assess the situation better enabling us to avoid the damages that stress brings it out. Mental disorder is one of the biggest challenges of societies around the world. One in for individuals is affected with some sort of mental instability which robs society of functioning and skilled individuals. It takes away the abilities of an affected individual to function correctly and go about doing their job and duties. The sooner this is recognized the better it is for an individual suffering from acute, routinely, and or chronic stress to find ways and solutions to this syndrome.

Unfortunately, most times, we are overpowered by the emotions that stress brings on to the point of being frozen unable to deduce solutions it is the time that we realize that we need help outside of ourselves to overcome these assaulting thoughts. Allowing distress to overpower a rational thinking basically limits, if not inhibits, the finding of a solution to the present problem.

The more alarming impact is not only how stress affects our physical bodies it also poses concern to our mental stability. There are a number of ways for a person who undergoes unrelenting acute stress to get help. Some of the more obvious available resources to us would be a support group that we can turn to in times of stress. Often times the mere fact that we can talk about what is troubling us to someone we trust, gives us a sort of release and relief from the factors that plague us and cost as stress.

Another way that we can get help is by talking to a therapist who can objectively assist us in identifying stress factors that set off the stress hormones in us. Therapist can help look at situations that cause you anxiety and can lead you to deducing if there is any validity in the fear that is overwhelming you. Medication in severe forms of stress can perhaps help with the problem, but there are better ways of dealing and handling stress factors without the use of pharmaceutical drugs.

Most experts would recommend mindfulness exercises so that a person can practice the habit of differentiating A real threat from supposed threat. Medication can sometimes switch off or switch on parts of your brain which need to function or not function at any given time. The problem with this is that our brains get used to the assistance of the drugs thereby making us reliant on pharmaceutical drugs to handle our stress. It does not build in us the ability to determine what reality is and what fantasy is. Mindfulness equates to being present at the moment and drugs will definitely work against that goal.

Check with your local community and find out if there are support groups that deal with stress. Knowing that you are not alone in your fight for control over your emotions often times make it easier for a person to understand that stress will happen, can happen and does happen. In addition to knowing this, a person will be better equipped in identifying how they can help themselves out of an emotionally charged situation by allowing them to rationalize and look for solutions instead of festering and worry and anxiety.

Find ways that will take you out of the stressful situation that is charged by emotion by doing things that give you pleasure like listening to music or painting a picture. Meditation has been proven to help realign the mindset of a person who is constantly under stress. Yoga is a good combination of mindful physical activity that engages your mind as well. Not only will the exercise make you feel physically better but it will also release a flood of dopamine to your brain, signaling relief and enjoyment.

Avoid anything that will give you temporary relief. When people are under stress the part of the brain that tells you to face or flee from a problem kicks in. To allow oneself to get clouded by drugs and alcohol exacerbates the situation even further. It may definitely give you a sort of temporary respite, but will not give you any long-term solutions to fend off irrational thoughts and crippling emotion later.

Chapter Eight: Child Stress

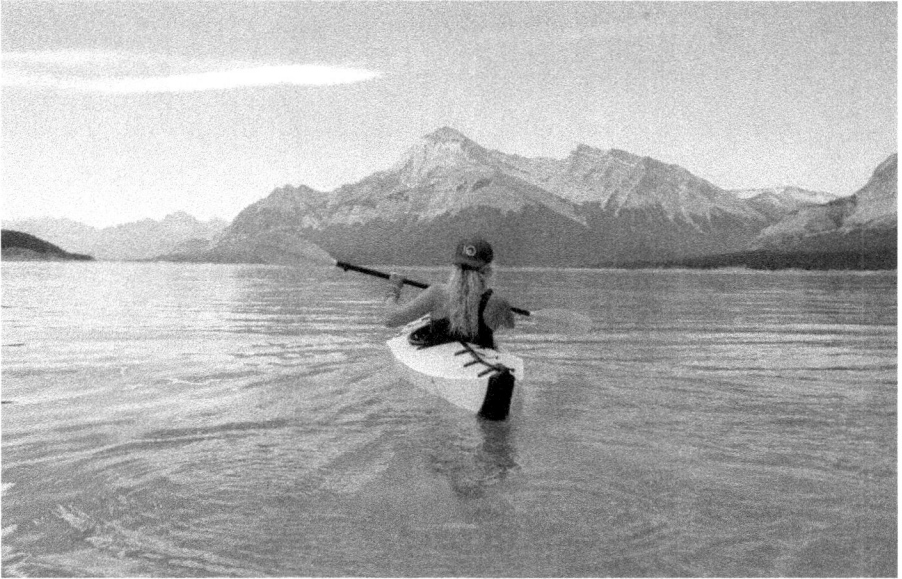

As adults we tend to think of childhood life as stress-free and happy. Perhaps it's because children do not have the same responsibilities as adults do. But that is in fact untrue if you think about it. Let's have you imagine yourself when you were a child. Can you think of times when you as a child had possibly some sort of stress but did not know what it was? Perhaps it was you transferring to a new school and not knowing anyone. It could be that your family had moved from one location to another. Or it could also be a disruption in the family dynamics that brought about the stress that you had felt as a child.

Children are not free of stress just because of their age. There are plenty of factors to cause a child stress and if you ponder on this for a moment look at the society around as you would realize that this is indeed true. We hear of incidences of bullying, we learn about the pressure a child is put through with academic demands. Sometimes it is the parents themselves to place stressful demands on their children which results to a highly strung child. These are just some of the impacts of stress on a child that is dealt by outside factors. As a child matures academic and social pressures create more stress for the growing adolescent.

What Happens When a Child Becomes Stressed?

When a person, in this case a child, is overwhelmed by pressures and stress that they are not able to communicate, it limits their creativity and inhibits their learning abilities and growing process. With the high demand of society to adults, so are children who are burdened with the same amount of pressure for them to succeed. If we were to get down to the nitty gritty of stress placed upon a child, we can look to two examples of a day in the life of young students from Korea and Sweden.

Did You Know?

Children in Korea start their long, academic day by attending school from early in the morning to late afternoon. When they are done with their regular school day, many of these young children head off to English classes which could last anywhere from 2-4 hours. They usually get home pretty late in the evening and have just enough time to sit down for a meal. When they are done, they head to their rooms to crack open books, do homework that needs to be submitted he next day, taking up about 2.5 more hours of their time. They usually go to bed late into the night, and wake up early the next morning to do the same thing over again. Because of the high expectations from them, they are often tired and burnt out by the end of the week. On the other hand, young students in Sweden go to school a little later in the morning as compared to their Korean counterparts, they leave school earlier, giving them time to spend with their families doing leisurely activities with no demands of homework to be done. The picture is painted pretty clearly and we get a good idea of where balance needs to be made.

Common Causes of Child Stress

Other times stress in children can be intensified by what is happening inside of the family home. Perhaps they overhear the troubles of the family, hearing arguments and knowing about financial difficulties that the family is going through. How can we help our children from being overwhelmed my problems that they should have no business knowing?

Children are perceptive human beings no matter how small they are. They pick up on the anxiety of the parents and begin to imbibe the worries of their caregivers. Be mindful about what you discuss with your children or in front of your children and most especially do not let on about problems that they have no business knowing. Another cause for a child stress could be what is happening around our community or in the world. Children are not usually able to express their emotions with words, therefore whatever bad news they hear on the television is absorbed and pondered on in silence. This could be a cause for unmerited fear and stress.

Make sure that they are not present for any programs on television that is only suitable for adult understanding. If it is absolutely necessary for a child to listen to the news be sure that you are there with them so that you can turn to them and explain what is going on.

Aside from the everyday stress of the demands of academics and peers be aware of complicating factors that could exacerbate stress in the child. Some of these factors could be an illness in the family, the death of a loved one, or separation and divorce of their parents. These events magnify stress factors of everyday life making it more confounding for a child to comprehend. Avoid having to make the child choose between one parent or another in the event of a separation or divorce. As tempting as it may be, do not expose your children to negative comments about your estranged spouse.

Develop a relationship with your child that gives your child the confidence to approach you at any given time, especially when they feel pressured or stressed by anything. Never undermine what is troubling your child by dismissing what they are feeling. Build in them a confidence in you so that they approach you when they feel a situation is oppressing them.

Symptoms of Child Stress

While it is not always easy to detect when children are under stress there are telltale signs and stress symptoms that will tell you that your child is under stress. These telltale signs could be changes in their sleep patterns or eating habits. Children under stress could display mood swings or they could act out through emotional outbursts. Children under stress can also have physical manifestations of the effects of stress in the form of headaches stomach aches or bedwetting. When a child is under pressure they have a more difficult time concentrating and learning. Another indication of stress in a child is social withdrawal. A usually outgoing child, if they start to spend time more by themselves, could possibly be undergoing some sort of stress that brings about confusion. Other indications of stress and younger children could be thumb sucking or bedwetting.

What You Can Do

To help your child reduce stress in their young lives make sure that you make yourself available for them. Create an atmosphere of confidence amongst the family where children can approach parents for anything and everything that they may be anxious or worried about. Listen to them, talk to them, and help them vocalize and communicate feelings that are within them. Sometimes just the mere presence of an available and open minded parent is enough to calm the child. Quality time is very important to building relationship that is based on confidence and trust. If our children know that they can approach us with confidence, they will be able to handle stress factors much better in their present lives and more importantly, as they mature. As parents we need to express genuine interest in the goings on in our children's lives in order for them to understand that they can rely on you.

There are times when we need to help lessen the stress and our children by helping them anticipate situations there by helping them prepare. One example would be letting your child know ahead of time about a dentist appointment. This is an opportunity for you to talk to them about what to expect when you get to the dentist. Keep in mind that a certain level of stress is normal tell your kids that it is OK to feel emotions like anger loneliness anxiety or fear that other people have those same emotions and feelings as well. They need to be reassured and they need to realize that you have full faith and confidence in them that they would be able to handle the situation and that they can always come to you for whatever it is that is bothering them.

Most of us parents have the skill set to handle talking to the child who is under stress. But what if your kid cannot or will not discuss their stressful issues? You may try talking about one of your own. This would show them that you are open to taking on difficult conversation topics and that you are readily available to listen to them when they are ready to talk. There are many children's books that are available these days that tackles difficult topics that cause stressful situations. Facebook's for children are aimed for them to learn how to cope with usual everyday stressors as well as unexpected and unforeseen events that may happen. Do recognize when it is time to get outside help in order to help your child deal with their stress.

When you notice that they're change in behavior persists or when the stress is causing grave anxiety or when the behavior causes significant problems that interact with their school life or with a life at home. As children grow into young adolescents, their stressors change as well.

Chapter Nine: Society and Stress

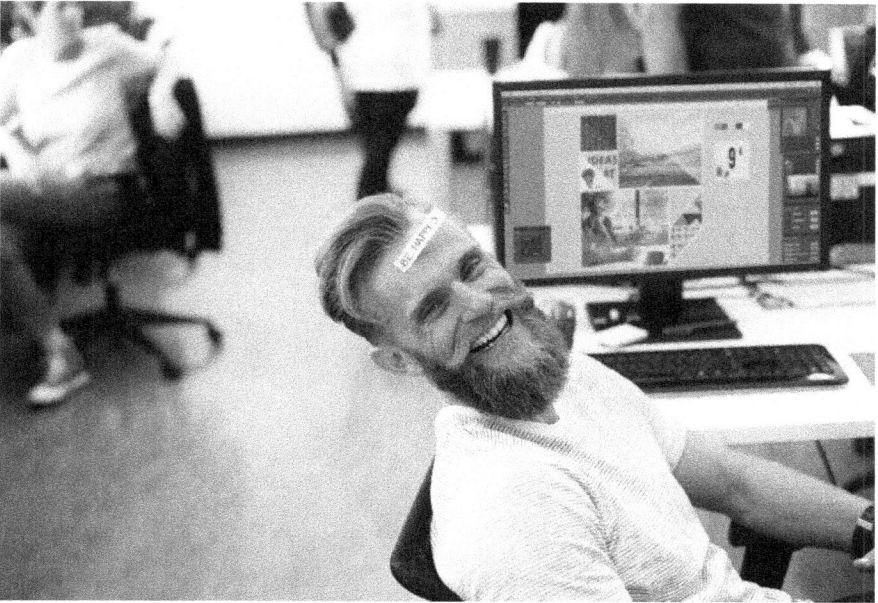

Another factor that causes us stress is the fact that we compare ourselves to higher standards. We worry about being good enough and if society in general will find us acceptable. Movies and television have somehow set the bar really high on what media perceives as beautiful. We look at what we have and compare it to what we don't have - more explicitly, we compare ourselves to others - and we figure that there is something inherently lacking in terms of what we should have, as dictated by standards set by a small minority of people with a far reaching audience.

It can be said that wanting to be the most popular, the handsomest, or the most beautiful is a difficult standard to meet because there will always be those who are better off, better looking, more talented, etc., than us. Perhaps when the world was younger in our mindset, when competition was not as big, it would have been easy to set such goals. But when we are "pitted" against billions of people in the planet setting those lofty goals is a recipe for discouragement and upset.

The pressures of society and modern life, along with the demands of responsibilities, career, and work can be considered as sources of tension undergone by people who face extraordinary situations, constraints, demands or opportunities. Some of these everyday pressures can lead to emotional imbalance which is collectively referred to as stress. But stress, doesn't always present itself as unpleasant. Take for example a willing, expectant, first time skydiver who would feel anxious about an upcoming jump as opposed to one who has no inclination to do it. They may both experience the same physical effects of the factors that release the stress hormones but both of them are assessing the situation using their own individual conclusions about how they are and will be handling the situation.

Adapting, the second stage after the recognition and assessment of a situation, is the bodily reaction wherein the intricate interaction of inner, physical and mental, systems could result in consequential effects to the person experiencing the demanding situation. They begin to feel stressed out and if this period lasts longer than a spell it could equate to more serious ailments.

Since the Stress affects us all differently, what may be a stressful situation for one may not bother the next person. There is no real bar to measure stress triggers which would apply to all because we are all made up differently and respond to stress factors in varied ways. There is no bar to set in terms of what would be considered stress for all. However, there are generalizations that can be made.

As discussed earlier, some of the most common situations of today's modern times bring about different forms of stress that can come from a variety of situations, emotions and events. With the ever growing pressures demanded of us by society, it is no wonder that more and more people are feeling on edge.

The physical effects of stress are undoubtedly a challenge people experience when under pressure. Keep in mind that stress isn't always a bad thing. If not for the chemical reactions in our bodies that would constitute a person to be considered under stress, human beings wouldn't have survived being a prehistoric animal's dinner. An advantage of stress is that it allows us to respond accordingly to a situation presented to us.

The problem starts when the stress experienced by an individual is prolonged. The effects of prolonged stress is not as simple as taking your mind off things. In the long run the effects against a person's health become more apparent and pronounced. These "minor" health issues could certainly escalate to more serious ailment.

An equally alarming side effect of stress is the mental anguish it can bring about, if not kept in check. The problem is, most people who are under prolonged stress will, by way of surviving the stress, adapt to the situation which ultimately becomes the "norm" for the person. It is very important that we unlearn how we operate under stress and learn to ask ourselves relevant questions about what is bringing about the stressors.

Stress and Gender - The Stats

Living in a society that is ever expanding coupled with the growing demands of personal life and society, women and men report having the same amount of stress levels. However, it is women who are likelier to report that their stress levels are on the rise with almost 50% of them reporting to have increased stress over the span of half a decade. Upon closer inspection, it is women who report more instances of their stress manifesting in physical and mental manners as opposed to men, although women are a lot better at making and maintaining important connections and relationships to manage their stress. There is also a reported difference of stressors between married women and single ladies.

There are reportedly more women, pegged at 79%, than men, who are quick to point out that finances is one of the factors of their stress. 68% of these women report that economy is another factor that increases their stress levels. 76% of the male population surveyed, on the other hand, report work to be a source of stress, with 65% of females reporting the same. 41% of the women expressed showing more physical and mental symptoms than men. 44% of the women report to go through crying bouts with another 32% who report stomach pains or indigestion.

Women are also more likely to be kept up at night because of their worries and stress. This is made evident by the 33% of women who report to succeed in getting enough sleep. 35% talk about the success they have in managing their stress. Although 75% of the women recognize the importance of getting the proper amount of sleep, only 33%

report success with their efforts in successfully managing the proper amount of sleep they should have. 64% women believe it is important to have a balanced diet, but only 36% of them report success in eating smarter and healthier. When it comes to physical activity and exercise to manage stress, 54% recognize this importance to curb or manage stress, but only 29% reported success in their quest for smart physical activity and exercise.

Married women also report of increased levels of stress than single ladies. Married women report of higher stress levels they suffer in a month as compared to those of single women. They are more likely to burst into tears, develop headaches and chronic tiredness. Women are likelier to cite relationships and family as important support systems they can count on during times of stress. They are also more likely to hold their friendships in high esteem as they figure that the friendships they keep help alleviate the pressures brought about by stress.

58% of the men surveyed agree that getting the right amount of sleep is vital to their stress management. Unfortunately only 25% of them are successful in achieving a proper night's rest. 59% of them understand the value of employing skills to manage stress, but only 30% of them manage successfully. While 52% of the men realize the importance of having a balanced diet and how this is crucial to their overall wellbeing, only 25% of them report having success with maintaining a sound and balanced diet. 52% believe in the benefits of being physically active and the bounties of exercise but only 26% of them are able to successfully and religiously carry out physical exercise.

Men and women who were surveyed reported various stress factors coming from all facets of their life, and both groups report of the different methods they employ to manage their stress. Generally, both men and women prefer quiet, sedentary stress buster activities like listening to music, catching a show or two on television and reading. Even a smaller number of both men and women report seeking out professional mental care. Women exercise less than men and give reason of being too tired.

On the other hand 34% of the male respondents reported exercising more than their female counterparts (23%) stating that it gives them something to do other than stress over a demanding situation. 29% of the men reportedly exercised to keep from getting sick. More women reported lacking the willpower to follow on through with professional advice regarding lifestyle changes to manage their stress. Many of the women realize that they lack the ability of exercise positive willpower in order to manage their stress.

57% women read to alleviate stress as opposed to the 34% of men who crack open a book to manage stress. There are also more women (54%) than men (39%) to manage stress by spending time with those they feel comfortable with, like friends and family. 27% of the women report that going to church helps with lowering their stress levels as opposed to the 18% of the male respondent who go to church in order to manage stress.

52% of the male respondents report listening to their favorite tunes as a way to alleviate or manage their stress as opposed to 47% of the female respondents. 21% of the males surveyed reported to resort to eating away their stress by way of food consumption as opposed to the higher number of 31% of the females. Almost half of the females surveyed reported to eat unhealthy foods or binge eat when under stress.

Symptoms of Stress in Men and Women	Number of Males	Number of Females
Anger or irritability	45%	46%

Lack of Interwst, motivation or energy	35%	40%
fatigue	39%	41%
Anxiety	36%	34%
Headache	30%	41%
Depression / Sadness	30%	38%
Stomach problems (indigestion, aches)	21%	32%
Muscular tension	22%	24%
Shift in appetite	19%	22%

Chapter Ten: Continued Research for Stress

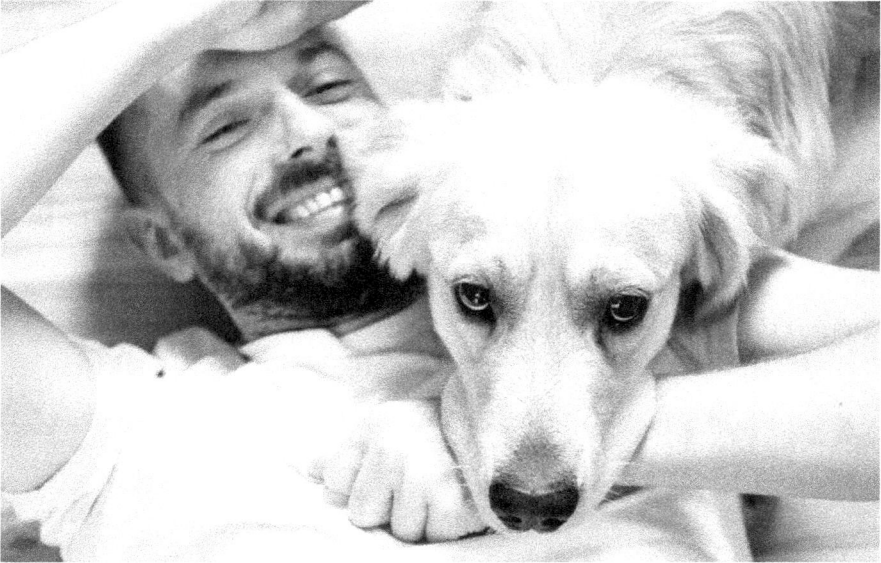

Stress affects everyone. No matter what age, race or creed, it is another thing that most of us have in common. The stressors of life are ever present, most especially in this modern day society we live in. The social hierarchy is one source of stress that researchers have studied and their studies have revealed that the social standing of a person in society has a correlation to the amount of stress experienced by an individual.

All of us feel stressed occasionally and some people cope better than others. An incident that brings about stress can be a passing occurrence or it could be something that happens over a course of time. All kinds of different stressors bring about health risks to an individual and the risks which have physical and mental impacts on an individual. Everyday stress can stem from the pressures of everyday, like pressures of daily responsibilities, school, work and family.

Stress also rears its head when a sudden, negative shift in our everyday lives occur, like getting fired from a job, separation and divorce, and illness. When a person suffers a traumatic experience like a horrible accident, a terrible assault on their person, war or natural disaster, the person who experiences any of these traumatic events undergoes traumatic stress. Individuals who suffer a traumatic event that shifts their routine and everyday lives usually experience and exhibit temporary signs of mental instability.

Most usually recover soon after the fact, but not all are lucky to have the support and assistance in their time of need. Some are left undiagnosed and confused about the damage they do not see happening to their psyche and are left with the burden of dealing the way they know how.

Long-term stress brings about a host of medical issues to the bearer of the stress which can develop into chronic ailments if not checked. When the stress is unrelenting or when the response continues after a threat has subsided, when your quality of life suffers, it is time to recognize that help is needed. The life-saving responses in our body like our immune system, our digestive system and our ability to get proper sleep is suppressed and interrupted by the stress that is being experienced.

A host of ailments like headaches, sleeplessness, irritability, anger, and sadness could be experienced by a person under stress. When a person suffers from chronic stress, these individuals are notably more prone to viral infections.

The symptoms of chronic stress become apparent over time, but harder to recognize is the effects of everyday stress, since the symptoms of routine stress is more relentless and the symptoms of chronic or traumatic stress, our body is not given the opportunity to return to the normal functions. As time passes, the continued strain experienced by your body may contribute to more life-threatening health problems like diabetes, heart disease, and hypertension. Other more serious, but unseen ailments, like anxiety and depression are the impacts of routine stress.

The first stress related disease discovered was the alarming increase of peptic ulcer. The gnawing and eating away at the stomach was the first ailment that was first thought to be strongly connected with the stress syndrome. The connection of stress and ulcers was the backbone of medical science decades ago but not too many were convinced. Australian researchers discovered bacteria that were present in ulcer patients, declaring that it was not stress but a bacterial infection that was causing the ulcers, overthrowing an entire field study on stress. When that theory was presented to the medical society, all ideas about stress management was thrown out the window with the advent of the creation of medicine to cure ulcer.

However, a few years later research took a sharp turn when scientists discovered that this gastrointestinal bacteria was not unique to those who had ulcers and that as much as two-thirds of the world population has it. So then the question begging an answer was 'why do only a fraction of these people with the same exact bacteria present in their systems develop ulcers?' Further studies were needed and that was what researchers did. Studies ultimately exposed that when a person is stressed the body starts to shut down all systems, including the immune system, the system in our bodies that has the ability to fight off sickness and disease.

It became apparent that when the immune system is shut down, the bacteria in the stomach begins to run amok. Stress not only diminishes the body's ability of self-healing, stress also inhibits the body to repair itself. If stress has the capability of undermining the immune system, then there must be more damage it can cause to a person. Stress hormones can trigger an intense cardio vascular response when a person is under stress.

The individual begins to experience shortness of breath, hard pounding of the heart and a spike in blood pressure. Stress and the flood of hormones increases blood pressure which damage a person's artery walls. Damaged artery walls become a repository of plaque, thickening the wall of the artery and constricting the flow of blood. When a cause of stress arises, when a stressor rears its head, the damaged artery is not able to expand; therefore, the muscle is prevented from being supplied with blood. When this happens for a prolonged period of time this can lead to a heart attack.

These are not theories or abstract concepts that can be placed in the back burner to be dealt with later. Proactive action needs to be taken now because stress has a silent but deadly manner of affecting the functionality of the body. Something has to be done in order to prevent further damage as soon as possible because, otherwise, stress will affect the health of an individual negatively down the road. Psychological and social stress can clog up the arteries, limit the flow of blood and jeopardize the wellness of the heart. And that is just the tip of the iceberg.

Research on stress reveals that stress can work in our body in a more sinister manner. Chronic stress or continued exposure to glucocorticoid, a stress hormone, can cause even more damage by destroying a person's brain cells. Studies on lab rats found that those exposed to stress had dramatically fewer brain cells than those of the rats who were not exposed to stress. What is alarming is that stress destroys the brain's hippocampus.

The hippocampus is the part of our brain which is responsible for our learning and memory. Stress can rob a person of memory and the ability to learn. Stress affects the brain in alarming ways. First of all, chronic stress can change the brain circuitry, which leads to the loss of capacity to recall things. Acute stress can lead to the troubling situation of not being able to recall what you, would've, normally known.

In addition to undermining our health, stress can just leave us miserable. The problem there is that if left unchecked and if allowed to fester, stress can lead to more serious problems that mess with a person's brain. Identifying the cause of the stress is an important first step to managing it. Determining whether the stress is real or supposed is a vital step in understanding the origin of the stress factor.

Stress and, pleasure are linked to the chemistry of the brain. When Dopamine, a neurotransmitter is released in the brain it attaches to receptors then signals pleasure. Those who have intact, undamaged by stress, brains, display the occurrence of dopamine which is the neurotransmitter that brings about joy, reward, and pleasure. When chronic stress becomes too overwhelming and kept unchecked, the hippocampus is not only duller, but the ability to experience pleasure is stunted as well. When the part of the brain that understands pleasure is damaged, it is difficult for a person to enjoy and appreciate the things that most others find joy. A beautiful sunset, a magical, mountainous landscape, a breathtaking work of nature's art is just not as exciting or compelling for the individual.

The correlation between stress and social standing is interesting one because mindset is really what matters. The saying "money isn't everything" can in fact ring true as there are many who are higher up in the social hierarchy of things that are not free from stress despite the availability of funds, whether for pleasure or self-preservation. When a person who has less than the rich individual has a mindset of success, no matter the outwardly depiction of reality, stress is better managed. Those who are lower on the social hierarchy have been observed to have different stressors that bring about the same health implications as those who are better off. This proves that, the stressors we all experience are different from one another but the outcome of the health impacts of unrelenting stress is almost identical.

People living in communities where safety is compromised on a regular basis have a lower expectancy rate of longer lives because they are always on the lookout; they are primed and stance defensively. It is within these communities where people produce high stress hormones which, over time take its toll. There is a price for exposure to chronic stress. Heart disease, diabetes and hypertension are just some of the more deadly, silent killers that originate from chronic stress.

Studies made in England revealed that stress, an individual's position in the hierarchy of society and how a put on weight, or the distribution of it, furthers the likelihood of developing life threatening diseases. People who are poised lower in the hierarchy of society and put on weight in the center of the body (the belly area) is known to have diseases that are linked to or originate from negative stress.

Fat brought about by stress and distributed around the middle of the body is much more dangerous than fat distributed elsewhere in a person's physique. It produces various sorts of hormones and chemicals and poses varied effects on a person's health.

Valuing stress reduction is very important for everyone, but our society today lauds doing more than is normal or healthy. Society has encouraged multi-tasking and gives accolades to those who seem to manage to work on more than one thing at a time.

Society has dictated that hours need to be filled in with numerous activities. From children, who attend school and then later has music lessons, football games, homework, or tutoring to adults running businesses, taking on multiple roles in the company, are admired by society. Our values have shifted radically. Early exposure to stress can leave lasting, lifetime imprints that are detected in the physiological and physiological health of a person.

Not only is a person's fat storage vulnerable when they undergo chronic stress, stress also has the upper hand on altering the brain chemistry and the capacity of a person to learn as an adult. Stress damages the ability of a person to react and respond properly to stressors, creating a vicious cycle of unrelenting negative impacts on their health, both physically and mentally.

It diminishes the capacity of the person to respond adaptively rather than maladaptive to stress. When chronic stress is left unchecked, a person is more likely to succumb to depression and they are more vulnerable to psychiatric disorders. People who have been experiencing chronic stress is more vulnerable to fall into depression.

Latest, groundbreaking research which keeps tabs on individuals who undergo stress as well as the cells of an individual reveals that stress can be traced even deeper in the body.

Taking the effects of stress down to the very basic machinery of how our body, cells and genes operate, studies have found that genetic structures called telomeres which secure and protect our chromosomes from thinning, corrode and degenerate by way of stress hormones. People have 46 chromosomes and each one is kept apart from each other by telomeres.

Telomeres, as we age, age along with us, but the interesting finding in people who undergo relentless stress reveals that the length of the telomeres in these individuals shortened drastically. This is a serious medical aging that needs to be put into light so that people can make a decision to take better care of themselves. This is a factual event that is not seen outwardly but is happening nonetheless. However there is hope. It has been observed that being able to talk about situations and events that cause stress can help heal a person's telomeres.

The question of what reduces stress and promotes healing was asked by researchers and the surprising answer was - compassion and caring, are some of the more important ingredients to the healing of a person who has been exposed to chronic and unrelenting stress. This is the mix that helps our cells to rejuvenate and regenerate.

Photo Credits

Page 10 Photo by user The Digital Artist via Pixabay.com, https://pixabay.com/en/stress-anxiety-depression-unhappy-2902537/

Page 17 Photo by user The Digital Artist via Pixabay.com, https://pixabay.com/en/brain-electrical-knowledge-migraine-1845962/

Page 21 Photo by user Mizianitka via Pixabay.com, https://pixabay.com/en/health-cure-vitamins-tablets-621356/

Page 27 Photo by user Graehawk via Pixabay.com, https://pixabay.com/en/alone-sad-f-depression-loneliness-2666433/

Page 35 Photo by user PublicDomainPictures via Pixabay.com, https://pixabay.com/en/ache-adult-depression-expression-19005/

Page 48 Photo by user TeroVesalainen via Pixabay.com, https://pixabay.com/en/men-women-apparel-woman-man-2425121/

Page 54 by user 5688709 via Pixabay.com, https://pixabay.com/en/hurry-stress-time-management-2119711/

References

5 Things You Should Know About Stress – NIH.gov
https://www.nimh.nih.gov/health/publications/stress/index.s
html

Basic Concept of Stress: Its Meaning &
Definition - Inflibnet.ac.in
http://shodhganga.inflibnet.ac.in/bitstream/10603/34682/6/06
_chapter%201.pdf

Have you ever felt lonely? - Stress.org.uk
http://www.stress.org.uk/ever-felt-lonely/

History of Stress - Humanstress.ca
http://humanstress.ca/stress/what-is-stress/history-of-stress/

Reminiscences of Hans Selye, and the Birth of "Stress" –
Stress.org
https://www.stress.org/about/hans-selye-birth-of-stress/

Stress – MedicineNet.com
https://www.medicinenet.com/stress/article.htm

Stress – KidsHealth.org
http://kidshealth.org/en/teens/stress.html

Stressed men are more social – ScienceDaily.com
https://www.sciencedaily.com/releases/2012/05/12052110402
6.htm

Stressed Men More Social? – ADA.org
https://adaa.org/understanding-anxiety/related-
illnesses/other-related-conditions/stress/news-and-research-
about-stre

Stress symptoms: Effects on your body and behavior –
MayoClinic.org
https://www.mayoclinic.org/healthy-lifestyle/stress-
management/in-depth/stress-symptoms/art-20050987

Stress Symptoms, Signs, and Causes – HelpGuide.org
https://www.helpguide.org/articles/stress/stress-symptoms-
signs-and-causes.htm

What is Stress? – Stress.org.uk
http://www.stress.org.uk/what-is-stress/

What's Your Stress Type? – HealthLine.com
https://www.healthline.com/health/whats-your-stress-type

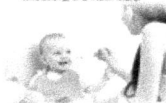

Feeding Baby
Cynthia Cherry
978-1941070000

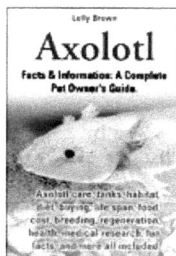

Axolotl
Lolly Brown
978-0989658430

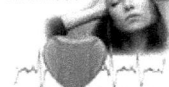

Dysautonomia, POTS
Syndrome
Frederick Earlstein
978-0989658485

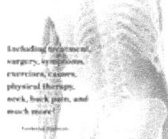

Degenerative Disc
Disease Explained
Frederick Earlstein
978-0989658485

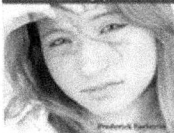

Sinusitis, Hay Fever,
Allergic Rhinitis Explained
Frederick Earlstein
978-1941070024

Wicca
Riley Star
978-1941070130

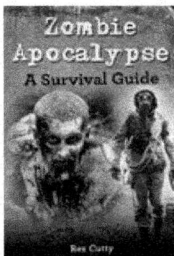

Zombie Apocalypse
Rex Cutty
978-1941070154

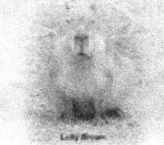

Capybara
Lolly Brown
978-1941070062

Eels
As Pets

A Complete Guide

Where to buy, species,
aquarium, supplies, diet, care,
tank setup, and more!

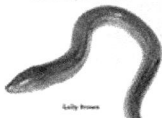

Lolly Brown

Eels As Pets
Lolly Brown
978-1941070167

Scabies and
Lice Explained

Causes, Prevention, Treatment,
and Remedies All Covered!

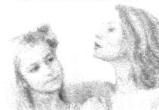

Information including symptoms, cure,
removal, eggs, home remedies, in pets,
natural treatment, life cycle, infestation,
rash specific, and much more.

Frederick Earlstein

Scabies and Lice Explained
Frederick Earlstein
978-1941070017

Saltwater
Fish as Pets

A Complete Pet Owner's Guide

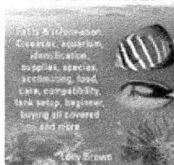

Facts & information.
Diseases, aquarium,
identification,
supplies, species,
acclimating, food,
care, compatibility,
tank setup, beginner,
buying all covered
and more.

Lolly Brown

Saltwater Fish As Pets
Lolly Brown
978-0989658461

Torticollis
Explained

A Complete Care Guide

Causes,
Symptoms,
and Treatment
all covered!

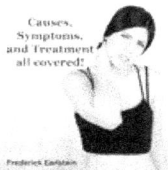

Frederick Earlstein

Torticollis Explained
Frederick Earlstein
978-1941070055

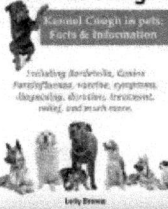

Kennel Cough
Lolly Brown
978-0989658409

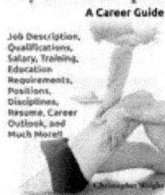

Physiotherapist, Physical
Therapist
Christopher Wright
978-0989658492

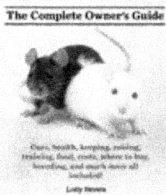

Rats, Mice, and Dormice
As Pets
Lolly Brown
978-1941070079

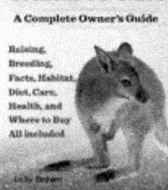

Wallaby and Wallaroo Care
Lolly Brown
978-1941070031

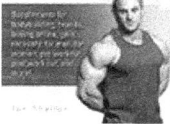

Bodybuilding Supplements
Explained
Jon Shelton
978-1941070239

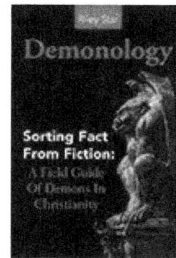

Demonology
Riley Star
978-19401070314

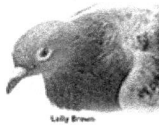

Pigeon Racing
Lolly Brown
978-1941070307

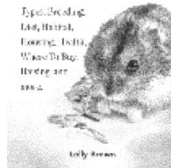

Dwarf Hamster
Lolly Brown
978-1941070390

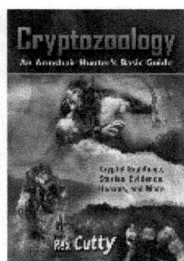

Cryptozoology
Rex Cutty
978-1941070406

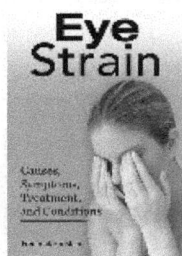

Eye Strain
Frederick Earlstein
978-1941070369

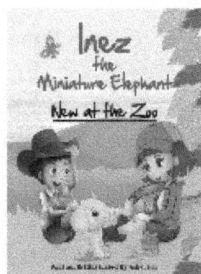

Inez The Miniature Elephant
Asher Ray
978-1941070353

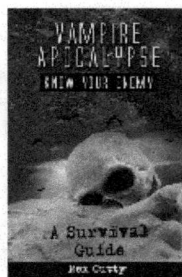

Vampire Apocalypse
Rex Cutty
978-1941070321

www.ingramcontent.com/pod-product-compliance
Lightning Source LLC
Chambersburg PA
CBHW071505200326
41519CB00019B/5879